Empath

Empath Healing Made Easy For Beginners (Handling Sociopaths and Narcisissists, Protect Yourself From Manipulation, Self-Aware Energy)

Kristine S. Everest

Empath: Empath Healing Made Easy For Beginners (Handling Sociopaths and Narcisissists, Protect Yourself From Manipulation, Self-Aware Energy)

Table of Contents

1 - Introduction

What Is Empathy?

Defined simply, empathy and healing may not readily form an association. However, there are many things that connect one to the other. To better understand this, let's begin by taking a closer look at each.

Empathy

This is a person's ability to understand and even share in another person's emotions, as well as feelings. Think of it as being able to put yourself into someone else's shoes and be able to experience their emotions as well.

Healer

This is a person who heals. These are people who are skilled in a particular type of therapy and are capable of treating different illnesses through various means. Some healers call upon divine help when working, whilst there are those who try to manipulate the body by engaging the mind and spirit.

Empathy and Healing: The Connection

Empathic people and healers share the ability to resonate

with others and tune into their energies. For most empaths, this can happen involuntarily. There are those who have more control over this ability, however.

What an empathic person can do, especially if they take it upon themselves to further their knowledge and improve this inherent skill, is to scan another person's psyche for their feelings or for past, present, and future life occurrences. Their heightened sensitivity makes them more adept at catching the smallest of changes in people especially in the energy they are emitting. In healing, energy is important.

Empaths can experience this towards their immediate family, their children, close friends, work associates and other acquaintances, their pets, the plants that they keep, and even with complete strangers. Some may even experience this towards inanimate objects in that they're able to sense its history. Empathy is not bound by time or space.

This is why some empaths can actually feel the energy of people from a distance. There are also empaths who are more in-tune with animals and are capable of communicating with them on a more profound level; think of The Horse Whisperer or someone like Cesar Milan, who can read the energies of the dogs he works with.

Healers and empaths also share a deep sense of knowing. They are more compassionate, understanding and considerate of others. A heightened sense of self-awareness is also common. Though there are also those who manifest these abilities even at a young age, but do not realize what they have until late in life. Some don't even realize it at all!

Empathy is inherited

Being an empath is genetic and inherent in our DNA as people. However, the ability isn't always developed in people. It can be studied and tapped into with consistent practice, of course. Empathy, itself, has both biological and spiritual aspects. Empaths can sense energy / emotion in differing ways as well.

2 - Different Levels of Being an Empath

As established earlier, there are many different kinds of empaths and they perceive the energy around them in varying ways as well. Here are the ten levels of empathy that people may fall under:

Psychometry

This is a person's ability to receive impressions, energy and even information from photographs, objects, as well as places.

Telepathy

This is a person's ability to read another person's thoughts. Most would be familiar with this as it has been portrayed in both literature and film countless times.

Physical Healing

This is a person's ability to actually sense any physical symptoms in another. In some cases, they would also have the ability to transmute or heal said symptoms.

Emotional Healing

This a person's ability to feel another's emotions; particularly, the deep ones that they may tend to hide. They are able to sense if someone is being weighed down by something and are also capable of helping with easing that burden.

Animal Communication

This is a person's ability to hear an animal's thoughts, feel their emotions, and even communicate with them mentally.

Nature

This is a person's ability to communicate with nature and plants. This includes allowing them to better tend to the ones that they keep.

Precognition

This is a person's ability to feel when something important is about to happen. You can think of this as that inexplicable restlessness that you cannot shake off.

Claircognizance

This is a person's ability to feel, knowing what has to be done given any circumstance. It is a kind of calmness despite being in the midst of chaos.

3 - Common Empathic Traits

Knowing

One of the first things you'll notice about empathic people is their ability to just "know" things even without having been told about it prior. It's a kind of knowing that is beyond what we often refer to as intuition or gut feel this is because their certainty and accuracy tends to be impeccable when it comes to this.

Needless to say, you'd have a hard time lying to one. The more in tune they become with their gift, the better they come at reading energies.

For an empathic person, being in a public space can be very overwhelming. Places such as stadiums, shopping malls, and supermarkets can fill them with different emotions often leading them to simply stay away. Remember, empaths are like emotional sponges and their sensitivity is far greater than that of the average person, therefore, they feel a whole lot more.

Describing an empath as a kind of emotional sponge isn't too far-off how they really are. The thing is that they feel other people's emotions and take those feelings as their own. This is why some of them tend to dislike the gift.

After all, can you imagine going through such a thing on a daily basis? It can be exhausting. Of course, this varies depending on how adept the empathic person is. For the most part, they will still feel people's emotions and this can affect them either negatively or positively.

Watching violence or anything tragic on the television can sometimes be unbearable for them. There are empaths who find it difficult to even read the newspaper as they become overwhelmed with emotion each time they do. This is something that empathic people cannot help.

They can easily tell whenever someone is lying or being insincere. There's that expression: "Ignorance is bliss" and for many empaths, this rings true. If a loved one lies to them, the pain they feel is double for they cannot help what they know.

It isn't just feelings that empaths can pick up from another person. They can also "absorb" ailments off of other people illnesses such as colds, infections and even body pain. This is especially so if the sick person is someone they love dear. The empath ends up developing the same symptoms as the other person. Think of it as something similar to "sympathy pains".

Physically, most empaths would also often have lower back problems, as well as digestive issues. This is where empathic people would be able to feel the emotion of another and in time, it begins to weaken too.

When that happens and it is left untreated, it can lead to stomach ulcers and IBS. Problems with the lower back tend to happen when the person is ungrounded or have no knowledge of even having the ability. There are ways of healing this, however, so don't fret. We shall get to those later.

They always look out for other people, particularly the underdogs and those who they know to be in emotional pain. They cannot help but feel drawn to them and given that empaths are capable of sharing these hidden pains, they also make for some of the best friends you'll ever meet.

That said, they also often become the people who others feel most comfortable opening up to. They have an always ready to listen ear, but the danger here is that if they aren't careful, those problems others may share with them can end up becoming their own.

They are almost, always exhausted. This is the inevitable result of them taking on too much from other people, whether it be voluntarily or involuntarily. Self-care is very important for empathic people, lest they end up burning themselves to the ground by absorbing too much, and too often from other people.

You may think that empaths, given their heightened self-awareness, would be much less prone to vices. However, this isn't true for everyone.

Many empaths tend to have addictive personalities; they are prone to developing dependencies on drugs, alcohol, and even sex. This is a way for them to block out the emotions they unconsciously absorb from others. Think of it as a form of self-protection, but a potentially harmful one.

Most empathic people are also drawn to various forms of healing, the metaphysical, and holistic therapies. For those who are aware of their abilities, they often find joy in healing others, but would often turn away from becoming healers themselves. Are there doctors who are empathic?

That is a possibility, but given the nature of the work and the environment some doctors are placed in, the likelihood is pretty slim. Of course, another reason could be that empaths are drawn to all things supernatural a doctor would be bound by the laws of medicine and science, something that empathic people might find too limiting.

They are very creative. From writing, singing, acting, dancing or drawing, most empaths would have a creative streak not to mention, a very vivid and extensive imagination. This could be attributed to the unique way they experience things; enabling them to have more insight and a deeper understanding of beauty as well.

Empaths tend to be nature loves and find that being in it is the best cure for their lingering feelings of fatigue. Most of them would keep pets as well and they end up forming very strong, familial bonds with the animals they care for.

Empaths love people, but all the same, they also have a deep need for solitude. They will always require their quiet time and this need does not change even with age. Both adult and children empaths tend to become moody or very restless if they don't get some time alone.

They tend to get distracted easily if they're doing something that isn't very interesting to them if it does not stimulate them enough. Boredom sets in very quickly for empaths as well and they are very prone to rumination.

It would be impossible for them to do something that they cannot derive any form of joy from. This makes them feel less authentic and as if they're not fulfilling their potential as people. In some cases, empaths do tend to get labelled as "lazy", simply because there's no way a person would be able to force them to do something they dislike.

So what catches an empath's attention? Typically, this involves the search for answers and knowledge. They are very curious people and many enjoy learning more about their ability and how it might be of better use to them, as well as others. They always have questions, but take it upon themselves to find the answer.

Are empaths timid people? Some are, some aren't. Most would be free spirits, however. They enjoy traveling and feeling every experience with intensity. These people are staunch advocates of living freely and saying yes to adventures that come knocking on their door.

You may think that an empath, given that they are prone to daydreaming and having rather chaotic minds, would be disorganized people, but this is not the case at all. In fact, many of them abhor clutter finding that it can actually block the proper flow of energy and only adds to them feeling weighed down.

Many empaths are intolerant towards a lot of things, this is one of the reasons why some people often find them either: too sensitive, too judgmental or simply hard to understand. However, being judgmental is far from what they actually are.

They simply cannot tolerate attitudes that most people simply brush aside. For example, they cannot stand narcissism and would often point this out as well out of consideration for the person, and other people.

An empath who is adept when it comes to their ability may also feel the different days of the week. Some would get something like a "Friday Feeling"; most of the time, this is what the collective around them is feeling. If everyone at work is excited, even if they don't show it or speak it, the empath would be able to feel that energy.

The same goes for negative energy as well; if everyone at work is feeling bogged down and then the empath would sense this and carry it around for the duration of the week or until the mood around them changes.

For empaths who are capable of reading energy from objects, it is likely that they would refuse or avoid buying vintage, antiques or secondhand items. Anything that has a residual energy which they can end up absorbing.

However, there are the curious ones who enjoy this; finding the experience to be like time-traveling as they get to "relieve" certain periods of time through an object and the energy imprinted upon it by the previous owner.

The same goes for empaths who can also sense the energy in their food. Some would refuse to eat any type of they meat as they can often feel the vibration of the animal (particularly so if the animal suffered in any way).

At first glance, most empaths would appear disconnected, moody, and aloof. Of course, this all depends on how they are feeling as well, but these people would never put on a mask to hide their emotions from the world. They are most prone to mood swings as this can be directly influenced by the energy they happen to absorb.

If they have taken on too much negative energy, they will

become very unsociable and appear miserable. This is because they refuse to pass on the negative energy to another person, but there are instances wherein others might misinterpret these actions as disinterest.

One of the biggest challenges an empath might face when it comes to forming relationships is trying to explain why they feel a certain way to other people. Not everyone would be able to easily understand how their ability works and there would always be those people who would even reject the very existence of it.

The latter is also one of the reasons why an empathic person might begin to hold themselves back, not wanting to be thought of as different and be treated as an outsider. Bottling up their emotions can actually be detrimental to an empath's physical and mental health. The more they do it, the greater the frustration they feel.

So, what can they do to protect and take better care of themselves?

4 - Being Empathic and the Ability to Heal

The gift of being empathic is certainly a blessing, but it comes with a lot of challenges. Imagine being able to sense the feelings, and even the thoughts of those around you. If they happen to be very positive then it wouldn't be that bad, right?

Now, picture the same thing happening, but with everyone's energies going in every direction. Happy, miserable, excited, nervous all of these things add up and can easily overwhelm an empath. It can make them feel physically ill, in some instances.

What if you had to go through that experience nearly every single day? What if you didn't really have anyone who understood your ability and would often misinterpret your actions instead?

It's quite sad, isn't it? This is the reality that most, if not all, empaths face. These things can easily cause them to detach themselves from others, preferring solitude as it is easier on them mentally and physically. However, that is no way to live, right?

This is why self-healing is important for empathic people. It is a way for them to detoxify and clear their head after a long day. After all, they get drained very easily of energy and would need to re-energize more often than the rest of us.

5 - What to Avoid if you are an empath

There is no doubt that withholding their emotions can be very detrimental towards an empath's health. The longer they do this, the more power these unreleased emotions and thoughts have. In time, they may become crippling.

If they aren't given the opportunity to express themselves honestly or are somehow withheld from it by another, this can result in a breakdown mental, as well as emotional instability which may manifest itself physically as well. Heart ailments are common in empathic people.

Aside from this, empaths should also try and limit their exposure to triggering stimuli. They can be very sensitive to TV shows that portray violence; particularly those that inflict physical and emotional pain to children, adults, and even animals.

Where some people would often cry, empaths can start feeling physically ill because of what they're being presented with. One of the main reasons for this is the fact that empaths do struggle to understand such cruelty and lack of compassion.

6 - Self-Care for Empathic People

Whilst there are things that can be avoided, there are plenty more that empaths have no choice but learn how to cope with. This is where the importance of self-healing becomes of value. There are many ways to do this, but here are a few everyday things that empathic people can practice in order to keep themselves from becoming drained by those around them:

Practice gratefulness meditation for at least twenty minutes each day. What this does is trigger the release of feel good hormones which would then balance out a number of stress hormones in our body. By doing this, you'd be able to regulate your heart beat and feel a lot less restless and anxious.

Make sure you get enough sleep each time. When you're sleepless, the mind is actually more vulnerable and the harder it would be for you to create a calm boundary around yourself. You also get more irritable which makes you more likely to start feeling negative energy.

Do manage your exposure to certain media properly. As much as possible, limit yourself when it comes to reading up on the day's news. However, if you'd rather not shield yourself when learning about world events (this matters greatly!), then make sure that you try and balance the negativity with something positive. Watch videos that make you smile or listen to music that calms you down.

Start decluttering your surroundings. Begin with the bedroom as this is where most people tend to keep things that mean a lot of them; if you find objects that carry unresolved emotional stories in them, do your best to start letting go.

Holding on to these can only increase negative energy around you and this is what you must seek to avoid. After you finish with one area, continue on and move to the next until you feel much lighter.

Do your best to avoid drama. This means that you should avoid people around you with are very gossipy. Do the same things with people who make you feel small and unwanted. Continuously hanging out with this kind of crowd can really bring your energy level down you don't need that. Protect your energy better and you'll really feel a lot lighter about yourself as well.

Whenever you start feeling overwhelmed to the point of exhaustion, always ask yourself: "Is this emotion mine?" For empaths, it is likely that the answer is NO. You are merely absorbing someone else's energy and feeling exactly the way they are in that moment.

Acknowledging this fact really does help when it comes to diminishing its effects. Once you understand that the energy isn't yours, you can begin to slowly detach yourself from it and restore your own. It might take a while, however, but meditation will certainly hasten the process.

Start learning how to say NO to people. The thing with empathic people is that they often feel quite guilty after saying no. Some would even feel as if it is their purpose to share some of the world's energy burden they want to fix things but want to avoid it simultaneously.

If you ever find yourself too overwhelmed to the point that you feel paralyzed by it; refuse and say no more. It is important to take care of yourself first before anyone else.

Spend some time outdoors. It needn't be somewhere far, like going into the mountains to camp. You can opt to go for short walks outside, especially if the weather is particularly good. Find a nice grassy spot where you can stand barefoot on the ground.

Do this for at least ten minutes a day whilst you practice

gratefulness meditation. By connecting to the earth, you are actually grounding yourself and renewing any lost energy. This practice has been proven to be very effective.

Make sharing joy and laughter a daily practice. Here's a fact: Laughing really does wonders for our physical and mental health. Do something that brings you joy on a daily basis. No matter how simple it is taking some time off to work on a hobby, treating yourself to your favorite food or spending time with people you love. It is important to step out of a negative frame of mind and change your routine a little.

7 - Energy Techniques for the Intuitive Feeler

Aside from the more practical ways that an empath can use to protect their energy, there are other more metaphysical techniques that they can use as a means of defending and stabilizing said energy. The idea here is to not shut out everyone else's energy. Instead one simply learns how to filter what they allow in. This also gives you more control over your ability.

To help you get started, here are two easy to follow techniques which you can practice whenever you feel the need to create a barrier between yourself and any unwanted energies in your surroundings.

The Zip Up

This one was created by Donna Eden. Visualize an energy cape or coat that you slip on in order to protect you against absorbing another person's energy this is what the Zip Up technique is meant to do.

Basically, it works with your central meridian, also known as the energy pathway which moves along the center line of your torso. This controls your central nervous system as well.

For many people, not just empaths, this central meridian often acts like a rod that channels the energy, thoughts, and feelings of the people around you. Whilst this is alright in some cases, you must also know how to properly protect yourself in order to avoid becoming overwhelmed.

In doing this, many empaths say that they feel more positive and renewed. They were also able to think with more clarity and tap into their own inner strength, shielding themselves from any negative build up in their environment.

To do it

1. Begin by placing your hand or both of your hands on the very bottom of your central meridian. This is loc-ated at the top of your pubic bone, facing up the body.

2. Follow this up with a deep breath, let go of any ten-sion in your body. As you do this, move your hands up the center of your body, all the way to your lower lip. You can also opt to do this with your hands touching your body or a few inches away from it. Try your best to focus on what you're doing and if you're distracted, pause then take another breath before

continuing.

3. You can repeat this practice for up to three times or whenever you feel as if it is needed.

Creating a Shield of Light

This one is meant to create a boundary between you and energy that you are trying to avoid. It will keep unwanted feelings and thoughts at bay, as well as help with clearing your energy field. This is particularly great for people who need more room to breathe, psychologically and energetically.

If you work in an environment where everyone's energies seem to bombard you all the time, this would be a great practice to do. It involves a degree of visualization so you might want to find a quiet space for this.

To do it

1. Begin by visualizing yourself being enveloped by a blanket of light. Imagine it wrapping around you like a shield, not quite touching your body but near enough. This is your own energy field manifesting physically. If you can, try to imagine what it feels like. Warm, cozy something that makes you feel very se-

cure.

2. Next, bring your elbows closer to your sides, keeping both palms facing outward. Breathe in deep and slowly breathe out as you slowly push both hands outwards; while you do this, visualize that you are spreading your light shield further as well.

   The more you can focus on this picture, and really feel it, the more effective this exercise will be. It will take a few tries, but with constant use, you will get the hang of it.

3. Remember that there is no need to rush this step. Go as slowly as needed. As you push outwards, visualize the shield of light expanding, the pressure of it against your palms, and how it's pushing away the energy that does not belong to you. Visualize all of the negative energy fading against the strength of your own light shield. Focus on that image as you breathe in and out slowly.

4. Follow this with a period of rest. Put your arms down comfortably at your sides and focus now on your breathing. Let the feeling of lightness fill you. Breathe

in and out slowly once more before moving on to your other tasks.

5. You can repeat this exercise whenever needed. However, it is best done in a place where you can have some quiet and without worrying about any time constraints.

Belly Breathing

As you may have noticed breathing plays a fairly central role when it comes to these exercises. This is because proper breathing can really help remove tension from the body and enable the mind to focus on the present.

Most of us have a tendency to breathe shallowly and rapidly, keeping it all in our chests. This is fine, but to reach that meditative state, you would want to breathe in deeply. For this, belly breathing is the best especially for the intuitive feeler. Why?

- It helps ground you, making you more in tune with your emotions and body.

- It helps center you.

- It can restore vitality, especially if you're feeling burnout.

- It can relieve anxiety and ease tense nerves.

Every chance you get, try slowing down your breathing and making sure that the air moves into the lower third of your lungs. You'll know that you're doing things right if your belly rises up each time you inhale and fall as you breathe out. There is a chance that you might feel light-headed, especially if this is your first time, simply return to your usual breathing pattern until you feel better again.

Once you do get the hang of it, try to incorporate breathing exercises into your daily routine. It need not eat up so much time; five minutes a day should be fine to center you again especially if you're going through a stressful time.

You can even do it while you're at work, at school, or even while you're out and anxiety starts kicking in. The bottom line is, this type of breathing is good for you physically, mentally and emotionally.

8 - Lifestyle Changes for Empaths

Aside from incorporating meditative practices into your daily routine, you can also opt to make lifestyle modifications which can help you maximize your gifts, whilst minimizing the energy draining effects it has on you. Here are a few simple ideas to help you get started:

Start with avoiding people whose energies are toxic to yours. There are those who will purposely manufacture drama in their lives and these are the people you need to stay away from. Try and keep your circle filled with upbeat friends, as well as people who are stable and optimistic.

Another thing you should avoid would be any form of media that affects you adversely. This includes books, unfortunately, as there are certain ones which can trigger ill feelings in many empaths.

It would be god to do a bit of research before purchasing a book or watching a movie this would help you avoid wasting money on something that you won't end up enjoying. Reviews would be very useful for this purpose.

As much as you can, spend plenty of time in nature. Plants are actually great buffers for your emotions and the environment immediately puts you in a more relaxed mood.

Treat yourself to getaways a bit more often, even if it's just a quick trip to the country or a garden close to your home.

Do not be afraid of doing things on your own. Most empaths recover better whenever they spend time by themselves. However, not everyone is very comfortable with this solitude. Think about the reason why you're not comfortable and do your best to get better acquainted with this side of you. Your mind will be thanking you for it.

Be more aware of the places you frequent that aren't good for your overall energy. This differs for every empath so a need to be more observant is needed. If you can, avoid these places. Explain to your friends why you cannot stay very long in that area, and suggest other ones that they might enjoy more.

If you explain your needs well enough, they should be able to easily understand the discomfort that being in that environment is giving you.

Be better at handling conflict. Conflict is inevitable chances are, you will never grow to like it. However, you can start managing it better. A counselor would be helpful for this purpose, but if you would rather try and provide a solution to the matter on your own, then there are plenty of self-help books that could give you more insight into it. Just research, you'll find exactly what you need in time.

Most empaths tend to choose professions where they can help other people think teaching, counseling, coaching, and healing. For empaths who are in these particular fields, it is important that you remember self-care.

Learn how to use your energy for yourself. Use the meditation practices previously provided, take some time off to restore your vitality put the same amount of care you give to others unto yourself. You'll be better at your job too!

Look around your personal space. Is everything organized? Is it clutter-free? A clean environment breeds a clear mind. If you can, always keep your surroundings organized. This lessens the amount of things you need to be anxious about and provides you with a calm place to rest your mind in. Remember, your home must be your sanctuary so treat it as such.

Here's a fact: Despite an empath's efforts to create limits between themselves and energy vampires, there will always be an "emotional hangover" that could happen. This refers to the residual energy left behind by a previous interaction.

Negative energy tends to linger a lot longer than others, often leaving an empath feeling ill or lacking clarity. In some cases, especially if an empath deals with energy vampires on a daily basis, it would take them a lot of time to recuperate.

So, what can they do in this situation? Well, cleanse themselves of the bad energy is a start. There are many different ways of curing emotional hangovers it really depends on the situation and what the person really needs as well. To help you better understand this and to give you an idea about how to cure emotional hangovers, here are a few strategies to get you started:

9 - Tips for Curing Emotional Hangovers

Shower meditation

If you have enough time during the mornings or during the weekends, use your time in the shower to help cleanse you of any negative energy that might linger. Stay under the shower head and the let water stream from the top of your head all the way to your feet; as this happens, recite the affirmation:

"This water will cleanse all the negative energy from my body, my mind, and my spirit." As you repeat it, visualize that bad energy leaving you. Repeat it until you start feeling lighter. By the end of it, you will feel a lot more rejuvenated.

In continuing with cleansing and adjusting your space to meet your needs, try using salt lamps as well as negative ion generators. What these would do is produce negative ions which then clears the environment of different pollutants such as mold spores, dust, pollen, odors, viruses, cigarette smoke and different types of bacteria.

Light a white-colored candle.

This is especially useful when you're meditation or simply unwinding after a long day. This creates a calming mood and also helps in removing negativity your surroundings.

Aromatherapy

Take advantage of the soothing effects that aromatherapy has. Rosewater is a favorite among many people, but choose the scent you feel most comfortable with. You can use sprays or synthetic oils which you'll need to add to diffusers in order to spread the aroma around. You can even choose purifying scents such as frankincense, myrrh and sage.

Nature

We've already established how effective being in nature can be if you want to ground yourself. Earthing takes this one step further and actually connects you to the ground first, take your shoes off and stand barefoot on the ground. Do this while your practice both visual and breathing meditation.

You'll find that focusing on nothing but the sound of your breath really helps clear the mind of any negative thoughts.

The earth, with its own natural energy, will replenish yours the longer you stay grounded to it.

Create your sanctuary.

If you live with other people, it is important to create a safe space for yourself. You'll need this if you want to properly meditate and keep any distractions at bay. It need not be an entire room. In fact, even a corner of your bedroom would work just as fine as long as it has the basics: incense, candles, flowers, and a totem that you can focus your gaze on while you meditate.

Now, when should you practice some of these tips? There need not be a "time" for it. These are basically small lifestyle changes you can add to your everyday life. Things that you can turn to whenever the emotional hangover becomes a little too burdensome for you.

As an empath, you'll find that this will happen a lot. So, instead of only acting when the problem arises, always be one step ahead and prepare for the situation.

10 - Empaths and the Workplace

Now, let's talk about the workplace. Sure, some empaths do have it easier than others are able to choose a suitable job for the empathic person. For the most part, the basic needs are simple it just has to be fulfilling and stress-free.

A job that maximizes their gifts is great too, something that many empaths would often go after. A job that provides them with an outlet for their quiet nature, creativity and intuition is highly recommended.

Some of the best careers for empaths would be those where they need to deal with only a few people. Most of them would be happiest in smaller companies or working from home where they have more control over who they interact with. Office intrigue isn't something that an empath would enjoy nor partake in.

Freelancing is also another option as it enables them to meet new people, but still have control over it. Flexibility in a job is a very important consideration, especially when it comes to time as they would need regular breaks in order to recover lost energy.

Many would choose self-employment for this reason, as it enables them to avoid the pressure of needing to deal with office hierarchy. If they can work within their own time, even better! Rigid schedules are not their thing and they perform better if they can work at their own pace.

There are empaths that do thrive in an office environment as well. However, this depends on a number of different conditions. For example, if the people surrounding them are all relatively positive this energy motivates an empath.

Which jobs are empaths drawn to? Well, whenever they opt to be self-employed, you'll find that empaths do excellent as editors, writers, artists, medical professionals, and any job in the creative field.

Other career options include: graphic and website design, accountants, lawyers with private practices, virtual assistants, independent plumbers and electricians all of whom are capable of setting up their own schedule.

There would be those who can even do well in business consulting and real estate; however, they need to be able to work at their own pace as well. Those with a keenness for nature would do well as forest rangers, landscape designers, as well as horticulturists.

As mentioned earlier, there are also those who prefer taking on professions wherein they can help other people. Many empaths often choose to become social workers, teachers, nurses, therapists anything that brings them closer to others in order to provide some degree of healing.

Some do well in animal rescue and non-profit organizations; all of which are very fulfilling jobs, something that an empath is drawn to. Of course, these are also careers that can be highly stressful, and as such, an empath would need to learn how to protect them from being consumed by work. Regular breaks would be necessary so they can refuel.

It is necessary for empaths to feel stimulated by the job they have chosen. Their skills should be put to use and their talents, maximized. Sure, they may not be the type to thrive in big corporations, professional sports, academia, the military, and government duties, but they can still contribute greatly to whichever career they decide to take on.

The thing with empaths is that they know themselves very well they know what they can do and how that can help. They are full of energy if they love what they're doing, if it is a job they're completely passionate about. For these people, money is just cherry on top of the cake. Their personal needs must be met first. Impractical, yes, but this is simply how these people function. Passion above all else!

Alright, now that we have possible careers outlined, let's talk about what are some of the jobs that an empath should avoid? Now, this doesn't mean that they would be incapable in these jobs. Rather, it only points to the high level of stress and energy demand that these jobs entails things that may not be healthy for an empath and may cause them to feel exhausted quickly. Many of these jobs also undermine their empathic nature.

One such profession would be sales. Given that this is a very extroverted job in nature, empaths might find it difficult to keep up. This is especially so if they encounter aggressive clients. Keep in mind that empaths, such as yourself, do absorb the energy from the environment you're in. If you encounter a number of rowdy people all day long, you will end up drained and burnt out.

The same applies to jobs in politics, public relations, as well as executive work where dealing with large groups of people is a constant. These are jobs that don't really require introspection or sensitivity instead, it's all talk and talk. Aggressively pushing products and ideas forward are things that empaths don't do too well at.

Corporate work is a big no-no for them. The mentality within the environment of big corporations can be extremely exhausting for empaths. These are places that do not give much value to an individual's needs and output is of great importance.

There is a rigid structure that must be followed; schedules, deadlines these are things that many empaths seek to avoid. Their lifestyle and way of thing wouldn't fit in well with it.

That said, there are certain times when an empath might not be able to avoid being in a job that they don't necessarily like. Everyone has to live and money is a factor in that, right? So, what can they do to improve their situation whilst taking advantage of their inherent skill? It's learning how to adapt to the environment. Learning how to read people can be important as well in order to avoid unnecessary confrontations.

To help with that, here are three simple techniques that you can try:

Observing Body Language Cues.

Research shows that words can only account for about 7% of how we communicate. Body language, on the other hand, accounts for about 55%, whilst voice tone comes in at 30%. Now, how is this useful? For empaths, this would be useful in determining if the person they're speaking to is genuinely interested in their conversation.

They can take certain movements as cues as to where they should nudge the topic towards. That said, this can lead to them becoming too analytical as well so find a balance. Instead of focusing too much on how the person is reacting, just stay fluid and relax.

Be comfortable and stay true to yourself. Do not try too hard to get the person to show interest nor should you feel bad if it happens that they are not always reacting positively.

Pay Attention to Appearance

Ask yourself, what is the first thing you notice when you meet other people for the first time? It is likely that you first pay attention to what they're wearing before moving on to any other feature. Are they dressed properly? Do they look shabby?

We tend to gather our first impression of someone based upon how they look. If a person is well-dressed, we immediately associate that with a healthy well being. On the other hand, if a person looks shabby then we tend to see them as unhealthy or someone who is untrustworthy.

Notice Posture

Another thing we unconsciously pay attention to is a person's posture. How confident do they look? Do they look shy or are they cowering as you speak to them? These are also keys to their personality as well as how comfortable they feel around you. Next time you speak with someone, observe where their hands are. If it's folded across their chest, this is a sign of defensiveness or wariness.

On the other hand, if their arms are comfortably placed somewhere around their body, in their pockets for example, then this means they're quite comfortable with speaking to you. People who are like this tend to be more open conversationalists as well.

Watch For Physical Movements

Observe the way people lean and the distance at which they do. The idea here is that people lean forward or towards people we like whilst we lean away from people we are not too fond of.

As mentioned earlier, crossed arms and legs are both signs of defensiveness. In some cases, they could also point to anger or self-protection. Another thing to look for is where people point their toes at most individuals would point their toes towards the person they feel most comfortable with.

Pay attention to people's hands

When people have their hands on their laps, in their pockets or behind their back, this suggests that they might be hiding something. Whilst this isn't always an accurate observation, it is stills something that you should try and pay more attention to.

Lip biting

Whenever people do this, it is their way of soothing themselves under pressure or after a rather awkward encounter/situation. The same applies to cuticle picking observe children who have a habit of doing this. They tend to be some of the shyest ones.

Interpreting Facial Expressions

Emotions can sometimes be easily read upon people's faces. Frowning suggests worry or overthinking. Pursed lips might mean contempt, anger, or bitterness. Crow's feet could point to the fact that this person is quite jolly, often smiling and simply easygoing. A clenched jaw, however, can signal tension.

Listen to Your Intuition.

It might take some practice, but you can develop the skill of being able to tune into someone's energy beyond simply reading their language and words. This is where your intuitiveness will come in handy. Intuition is what your gut feels as opposed to what your head says.

Bear in mind that there is a difference between the two. This is the nonverbal information which you perceive through images and not by logic. If you truly want to understand a person, what really counts is who they are inside and not their outward appearance. Your intuition enables you to unravel the depth to a person one which others may not be able to easily see. This is your gift, after all.

Checklist of Intuitive Cues

Trust your gut feeling. When it comes to first meetings, listening to your gut is key given your gift of being able to feel people's energy. For most empaths, a first meeting is more than enough for them to be able to tell if they would be able to comfortably spend time with a person or not.

In fact, some of them can have a visceral reaction to negativity, allowing them to steer away from a potentially harmful friendship. So, listen to your gut feel as this serves as your internal truth meter.

Pay attention to how your body reacts to certain interactions. In particular, observe whenever your goosebumps rise up. These are physical manifestations of energy and can be great intuitive signals that can convey information when it comes to how people move us. They tend to happen during moments of some importance, whether we realize it or not, so be more aware of their appearances.

Have you ever had an "aha!" moment? Now, for most people, they may dismiss this as nothing of value, but for empaths pay more attention whenever this happens. These are moments that could provide you with great insight into the person you're speaking to or simply the current environment you are in. These things tend to happen in a flash, however, so if you're not very alert then you can easily miss it.

As mentioned earlier, some empaths are actually capable of physically feeling another person's symptoms and emotions. Think about it, whilst you're reading people, have you ever had stabbing pain somewhere in your body?

Did a meeting with someone leave you with a tingle and an unshakable positive feeling? Speak to the person you're with, ask them if they're feeling any pain this is how you'll be able to confirm if this is a result of your empathy or something else entirely.

Sense Emotional Energy

Emotions are an expression of our overall energy. This is the vibe we give off to other people and the same ones they project onto us. Have you encountered people who simply feel really good to be around with? The energy they give off is full of vitality and they can easily improve your mood.

On the other hand, you have others who can be draining and make you want to move away from them. As subtle as these energy projections are, empaths can easily pick up on them given their inherent sensitivity to it.

11 - Strategies to Read Emotional Energy

Sense People's Presence

Presence refers to the overall energy that we emit. This, however, isn't always related to their behavior and words. Imagine it as something that surrounds people like a cloud over their heads or a light around them. It's the atmosphere that they carry around them. Ask yourself this: Does the person you're speaking with have a friendly presence? Are they colder or distant?

Watch people's eyes

There is a reason why people say that the eyes are the windows to our souls this is because they can also transmit powerful energies. Just as our brains have electromagnetic signals that can extend beyond our body, there are studies that show how they eyes have this as well. So, when you're reading people, take some time to observe their eyes.

What kind of energy is it giving off? Understanding? Caring? Angry? Some empaths can sense whenever a person's guard is up by simply looking them in the eye. They can tell if the person is burdened by something or if they're hiding something heavy in their souls.

Notice the feel of a handshake, hug, and touch

Pay more attention to how a person's touch, handshake, and hug feels. We all share emotional energy by means of physical content; it can be comparable to a subtle electrical current. So, if you're meeting someone new, observe how physical contact with them makes you feel.

Is the handshake comfortable? Did it leave you with a feeling of warmth? Or did you feel shaken by it? Did the other person appear confident or timid? These are a few important key points to keep in mind.

Listen for people's laughter and tone of voice

A person's tone and the volume at which they speak can signal a number of things about their emotions. This is because sound frequencies also create vibrations. Observe how people's tone affects you whenever they speak. Does it feel soothing? Abrasive? You can learn of a few things about how they might be feeling at the given moment or how they feel about you just by listening to how they speak.

12 - The Connection Between Diet and Empathy

Do you tend to experience digestive issues often? IBS or an upset stomach? Are you sensitive when it comes to certain foods? Do you tend to have an aversion towards smoking, drinking alcohol, and taking prescription drugs?

If you answered yes to most of those questions don't fret. These are actually common things that many empaths tend to experience. Think about it: you process the energy you absorb through your energy centers, which are some of the most subtle parts of your body.

Every single day, you go through this, and the energy you absorb won't always be positive. In time, it all accumulates, and gets integrated into your system. This often leads to issues which can manifest physically as symptoms of various illnesses.

So why do empaths have sensitive bodies, and systems?

For the most part, this can be attributed to an actual lack of information about what is good for an empath and what they ought to avoid. Health and fitness aren't always top concerns for empaths, as they focus more on their mental health instead. However, as we've already established, every aspect of our body and self is interconnected.

Most empaths tend to abuse their bodies, eating and doing things which are detrimental to their overall well-being. Some turn to food as a means of comforting themselves after a challenging day, others might even use alcohol as a way of turning down the overwhelming feeling within them.

This, however, is the wrong way of doing things.

Empaths must learn how to better care for their health and how to strengthen their bodies. A strong body equals a strong mind both things that you need in order to overcome many of the challenges that come with your gift.

Just as much as you listen to other people's worries and problems, you must also learn how to listen to your own body. Listen to your system. Tune in to the subtle signs that your body is giving you and start doing things that would boost its overall health.

Did You know that eating the right food can keep your mind healthy as well? You eat certain food to improve your heart health, lower the risk of diabetes, and certain cancers but were you aware that the same can be said for improving your focus, memory, and overall brain function?

A few simple dietary changes can make you less susceptible to mood swings and help you focus better. There are food items that can lower anxiety and help you avoid falling into depression.

Remember, what you eat can also affect how your brain functions so always include brain-boosters in your diet. Here are a few examples of what you should routinely have:

Fatty Fish

An average person's typical diet would often lack important omega-3 fatty acids and is, instead, high in trans and saturated fats which are known to produce negative effects on the brain.

Consider the fact that or brains are largely made up of fat, and the fact that the body cannot manufacture its own supply of essential fatty acids, then it only goes that we need to rely on a daily supply of omega-3 fatty acids in order to meet our needs.

Whole Grains

When it comes to brain fuel, our primary source for this would be glucose which comes from carbs. However, it is of importance that you choose complex carbs for this as simple carbohydrates are known to actually create spikes in our blood sugar level. Healthy sources of glucose include whole wheat products, oats, bulgur, wild rice, soy, beans, and barley.

Lean Protein

Next to carbs, protein is another substance that's abundant in our bodies. Tryptophan, a building block of protein, actually influences our moods by helping produce serotonin. Now, for the unfamiliar, serotonin is commonly referred to as nature's Prozac and is also well known to help curb the effects of depression.

Some of the best lean protein sources available include eggs, chicken, beans, fish, and turkey. These would help keep serotonin levels in the body properly balanced. Coupled with complex carbs, they facilitate the flow of tryptophan into the brain, helping reduce the symptoms of anxiety, depression, and improves overall cognitive functions.

Leafy Greens

Alright, so veggies aren't exactly everyone's favorite but after you learn of their benefits, especially fr your mental health, you might change your mind about excluding them from your diet. Let's start with the basics these leafy greens are high in folic acid. Now, why does that matter?

Well, any deficiency in folate, as well as other B vitamins, is actually associated with depression, insomnia, and fatigue. As an empath, these are three things that you need to avoid at all costs.

Selenium is also another important component when it comes to relieving the symptoms of fatigue and anxiety. This can be readily found in broccoli as well as walnuts, onions, chicken, seafood, and brazil nuts.

Mood Foods: How Amino Acids Feed Your Brain

We've established the importance of getting a sufficient supply of amino acids to the brain, but not quite how it helps in boosting its overall functions. The four key mood chemicals, also known as neurotransmitters, are made up of amino acids. Protein-rich foods such as fish, beef, chicken, and eggs contain all twenty two types of amino acids.

Now, including these into your daily diet can help with:

- Boost your mood

- Kick starting the brain's repair job

- Frees you from cravings which sometimes results as an emotional response

It might seem as if restoring depleted brain chemistry is too big of a job for a single supplement, but you'd be surprised to know that this isn't the case. This is because three out of the four neurotransmitters that significantly affect your moods is comprised of a single amino acid each. Biochemists have successfully isolated these key amino acids, allowing you to add the ones you specifically need to your diet.

Studies confirm the effectiveness of using these targeted amino acids to help increase the amount of neurotransmitters in our body which, in turn, helps with eliminating depression, lowering anxiety levels, as well as decreasing cravings for alcohol, food, and even drugs/medication.

13 - Restoring Energy and Focus

One of the biggest things that empaths tend to struggle with is the lack of focus and the fact that their energy gets drained very easily; this is especially so if they are surrounded by negativity and their brain is inadequately fueled due to a bad diet. This makes them more vulnerable, so to speak.

Sure, a shot of caffeine can help, but too much of it can also be bad. Why not turn to something more natural then? L-Glutamine is often referred to as such. It is an all-natural brain stimulant that serves as a very potent brain fuel.

Without it, you will feel slow and have a harder time trying to focus and filter out any unwanted energy. It would also be harder for you to stay on track mentally this leaves many people feeling lethargic, which also puts them at risk of slipping into depression.

For empaths, making sure that your diet has plenty of this natural caffeine will be beneficial. Not just for your interaction with the people around you, but for being more productive when it comes to work as well.

Boosting Your Ability to Relax

Another thing that many empaths struggle with would be relaxing. One would think that after a long, tiring day of dealing with people, empaths would find it very easy to unwind and get into a more relaxed state of mind. However, this isn't always the case.

This is where GABA or Gamma Amino Butyric Acid enters the picture. Think of it as a natural valium which acts like a sponge, absorbing any excess adrenaline along with other by-products left by stress.

It is capable of draining the stiffness and tension out of our muscles, and is also known to help with smoothing out seizure activity in our brain. In fact, it is also given to heroin addicts who are going through severe anxiety following detoxification.

Needless to say, it is very effective when it comes to diminishing stress levels in the body and enabling empaths to feel more at ease.

Food vs. Comfort

It's no secret that there are people who use food as a means of comforting themselves. Some find that it produces drug-like results, allowing them to forget their worries for the time-being.

Many empaths are prone to this particular problem, using food to make themselves feel better. Food can often compensate for the depletion of endorphins in the body, something that affects empaths more than the average person.

Think about it this way, what they go through on a daily basis can seem intolerable after the effect of these endorphins fade. Food becomes a secondary source for it, however, and thus many turn to it. This results in overeating just to feel that temporary "high".

If you use food in this manner, you are using them in the same way as synthetic drugs. While this might seem harmless at first, the way it can adversely affect your health is a very real problem. It is addictive in the same way cocaine or heroin is, and can be just as damaging if not controlled.

Ask yourself, do you often find yourself wanting to eat more after an overwhelming day? Do you tend to pour out your feelings but binging on your favorite food?

Some people will treat this lightly even make a joke out of

doing it. However, it can become a real problem especially for empathic people who then start becoming dependent on the "feel good" effect that food has on them. Once that fades too, what happens? The crash happens.

Fortunately, nature provides us with safer alternatives.

Serotonin, the All-Natural Prozac

Did you know that one of the easiest deficiencies that people can develop is low serotonin levels in the body? This is a rather jarring thought given its function to make us feel good, content, and energetic. So, how does this happen? It really all boils down to the kind of diet we have.

There are very few foods that contain Tryptophan, the amino acid that enables the body to produce serotonin. If you're dieting, you're already at risk of developing low serotonin levels. It can also be genetic some people are simply preconditioned to have low amounts of it. Stress is yet another trigger for its decline, often making it fall to amounts so low that it can set off a number of emotional disturbances.

In fact, restoring proper levels of serotonin in your body can become a life or death matter. Again, empaths are most prone to this, but even the average person can experience its ill effects. Violent crimes and suicides are also closely associated with serotonin deficiency. The same applies to fatal obsessions, anorexics and the self-hate that bulimics experience.

For some people, it can be difficult to understand that symptoms such as fear, low self-esteem, and the need for control are all biochemical problems and not solely psychological ones. However, the use of Prozac and its success gives us insight to the more biochemical nature of these issues.

14 - Inspiring Change by Using Your Empathic Abilities

Cultivate Your Curiosity

It is inherent in empaths to be very curious about people. Some can find it quite easy to strike up a conversation with someone seated next to them on a bus, and be able to find simple connections that make the exchange beneficial for both people involved.

This is because empaths have also retained that inquisitiveness which came naturally to us as children, but one which society has all but erased in most others. This is also why some people tend to center the conversation on themselves, finding their own person more interesting than other. Empaths understand this on a deeper level.

The thing that's great about curiosity, whether you're empathic or not, is the fact that it truly expands your empathy towards others. You can learn plenty through it. You can encounter lives, stories, and people whose views are vastly different from your own.

It can open your eyes to something much bigger than yourself; this can become the key to happiness as well. By open-

ing up your perspective, you start seeing that all your worries were for naught.

Cultivating curiosity is something that you slowly work
yourself up to; yes, not every empath is capable of striking
up a conversation out of the blue. For some it takes time.
Try starting small.

Chatting about the weather can eventually move onto other
topics, and help you understand the person you're speaking
to. Think of people as stories, each one is different, each one
is colorful. You simply have to turn the page and learn more
about them. Connect with people.

Remember, in conversing, you must know how to listen and
how to open up.

Step Into Someone Else's Shoes

Walk a mile in someone else's shoes before you judge them.
Isn't that how the popular saying goes? Most people would
find this difficult as there are many things that prevent
them from empathizing with another.

For some, it's self-centeredness, and a belief that they are superior. For others, it's simply disinterest. Empaths are great at this, however. People like you are gifted with the ability to actually live another person's life.

Think deep-sea diving is an extreme sport? Well, what if you can gain a direct experience of it through others by making use of experiential empathy? Yes, it is one of the most challenging types of empathizing with others. However it is also one of the most rewarding depending on how you use it and on what.

Impossible? Not quite. Take George Orwell for example. After spending years as a colonial police officer in British Burma, he went home to Britain, absolutely determined to experienced what it was like for people who lived on the social margins.

He wanted to submerge himself, to discover what it was like for them. And that he did dressed as a tramp with a tattered coat and worn down shoes, the author lived on the streets of East London alongside vagabonds and beggars.

The result of which is what we find recorded in his book: Down and Out in Paris and London.

The experience brought about significant changes in his priorities, beliefs, and relationships. It opened his eyes to the fact that homeless people were not "scoundrels" as the rest of upper society would label them. Instead, he developed new friendships, gathered great material for his work, and radically changed his views on inequality.

In this manner, he was able to turn his empathy into something powerful, something that could inspire change not just within him, but to those around him.

Observe! Be more open to different experiences the more you open your eyes to the things you would have avoided, the more you'll learn about the world around you and your part in it.

Inspiring Social Change

Turn your weaknesses into strengths. Yes, being empathic is difficult, but there's also great strength in it. With a person's ability to empathize, the world would be in shambles; history's greatest movements would not have happened and we will be stuck in a world of barbaric beliefs where brute strength rules over the weak.

A good example of this would be the movements against slavery which began in the 18th and 19th centuries, on both sides of the Atlantic. It was a time when abolitionists put their faith, not in sacred texts, but in human empath. They did what they could so that people saw and understood the suffering within the slave ships and the plantations.

The International Trade Union also blossomed out of empathy between the workers who were united by their shared exploitation. That is strength.

More recent events such as the Asian tsunami of 2004 showed the way in which empathy can bring an entire world together to help the response was overwhelming, with even the poorest of nations providing what they could to those in need. That is strength. It helped with healing the wounds left by the event, it helped peopled find their way again.

Can you imagine living in a world where empathy does not exist? A world where it is frowned upon and hidden?

As difficult as it can be living as an empath, you must also recognize your own strength and how you can contribute to the whole. Whether it be by individual deeds or a collective effort, it is important that you recognize what you can do.

Acknowledge the gift and believe it is such.

Once you see yourself as something of value, healing would happen naturally. After all, the only way you can really help others is if you're capable of taking care of yourself first and foremost.

Thank You

As we reach the end of this book, I want to say thanks for reading this book.

I want to get this information out to as many people as possible. If you found this book helpful, I would greatly appreciate you leaving me a review. This helps others find the book as well.

Disclaimer

This document is geared towards providing exact and reliable information in regards to the topic and issue covered. The publication is sold on the idea that the publisher is not required to render an accounting, officially permitted, or otherwise, qualified services. If advice is necessary, legal, financial, medical or professional, a practiced individual in the profession should be ordered.

This information is not presented by a financial or medical practitioner and is for entertainment, educational and informational purposes only. The content is not intended as a substitute for professional medical advice, diagnosis, or treatment. Always seek the advice of your physician or other qualified health care provider with any questions you may have regarding a medical condition. Never disregard professional medical advice or delay in seeking it because of something you have read.

The information provided herein is stated to be truthful and consistent, in that any liability, in terms of inattention or otherwise, by any usage or abuse of any policies, processes, or directions contained within is the solitary and utter responsibility of the recipient reader. Under no circumstances will any legal responsibility or blame be held against the

DISCLAIMER

publisher for any reparation, damages, or monetary loss due to the information herein, either directly or indirectly.

Last Updated: 11.Jul.2017